PROSTATE CANCER:

A FAMILY AFFAIR

Proactively Addressing Prostate Cancer
Has Reduced Our Chances of it Becoming
Our Death Sentence

Thomas A. Butts, Jr.
Derrick A. Butts

Publisher's Note

ISBN 9781705398340

Limit of Liability – Parts of this book were taken from Internet/web sources. The web references at the end of this book were active links and correct at the time of publication but may be subject to change.

Cover design and layout by Kristopher M. Mosby

Edited by Melinda Ruben

DISCLAMER

This book is for information and inspiration only. It is not intended to be medical advice. My son and I are not physicians, and we have never worked in the medical field. My purpose is to share my family's experiences. We are survivors and there is life after prostate cancer.

Every situation is unique, but we can certainly benefit from the experiences of others. As you consider any of the suggestions presented in this book, please consult your physician.

Thomas A. Butts, Jr.

TABLE OF CONTENTS

DEDICATIONS

Because of their continued support and devotion, I dedicate this book to my sons, Derrick, Steven, and Karlton. They all have accomplished great things, and I am a very proud man.

In addition to being service-oriented, good men, they have excelled academically and professionally. Derrick and Steven each hold master's degrees, and Karlton has a juris doctorate. I pray for their continued success and that they will achieve every goal they set.

I also dedicate this book to the memories of all men and their loved ones who have lost their fight to prostate cancer.

PREFACE

There are three important steps to improve cancer survivability:

(1) Early detection
(2) Proper treatment
(3) Frequent follow-ups

I wrote this book to share my family members' experiences with prostate cancer. My primary purpose is to describe what we did to increase our chances for longevity post-surgery.

I was diagnosed in 1994 at age 59. My brother Carl was diagnosed in 2005 at age 67.

My father, Thomas Butts, Sr., also lived with prostate cancer. He didn't discuss his diagnosis; we learned of it after he passed away in 1995. He chose no treatment and subsequently passed from an unrelated condition.

My sons and grandsons are well aware of our family history and the likelihood they may be impacted. They are prepared.

When I began writing this book, my oldest son Derrick was already diagnosed (at age 53) and treated successfully for prostate cancer. He shares his experiences in Chapter 10. Derrick has two young adult sons, and they too are aware and prepared to be proactive.

Challenges of all sizes and types arise each and every day. I believe the most important thing is to deal with them in the manner that is best for you and your family. With so many resources available today, finding information about prostate cancer is much easier now than when I was diagnosed in the 1990s. However, physicians urge caution since there is an equal amount of misinformation.

Advances in medicine have made a tremendous difference in how cancer is detected and treated. We owe it to ourselves to learn as much as possible and share knowledge since the prevalence of prostate cancer is higher for some demographics than for others. Let's do our part to prepare future generations.

This is my second book. My first book is entitled:
"AMAZING BENEFITS IN TRAVELING ON SOMEONE ELSE'S
DIME." It is available at: amazon.com and barnesandnoble.com. Search
by author or title. ISBN: 978-1-4269-4224-2 (SC)

That autobiography focuses on my life from early childhood through
2008. It shares how I became a licensed pilot at age 16, flew several types
of aircraft, and survived a major fire aboard an aircraft carrier where 51
men died.

During my 40 years of military and professional service, I traveled to 16
countries and chronicled my experiences.

I'm also working on my third book, "INSPIRATIONS OF THE HEART,"
a collection of romantic poetry. The poems were written and inspired by
women I met.

ACKNOWLEDGMENTS

I want to thank my son Derrick for sharing his experiences with prostate cancer with me.

Also, thank you to my wonderful girlfriend, Miss Sylvia W. Johnson, for her love and consideration during the time I was writing this book. I incorporated many of her suggestions. Sylvia has been very loving and caring and has brought much joy and happiness to me in these my twilight years.

Thank you also to Stan P. and Jamie V., who are prostate cancer survivors, and Melvin B., newly diagnosed with prostate cancer, for taking time to review and provide valuable feedback on the content, flow, and impact of our book. They share my desire to be helpful to others.

INTRODUCTION

I believe life is a quest for survival, with myriad daily challenges. I also believe the most important asset we have is good health, and that we should do whatever we can to maintain it. The medical community advises an annual physical examination, which can uncover small problems before they become big and unconquerable.

This certainly applies to prostate cancer. If it is detected early during a physical examination, you can **focus not on what happened to you, but how you can and will deal with what happened to you.**

"Prostate Cancer does not have to be a DEATH SENTENCE." In 2019, the National Cancer Institute (NCI) estimated the number of new cases of prostate cancer to be approximately 174,650, which is 9.9% of all new cancer cases. The number of deaths from prostate cancer was estimated to be 31,620, which is 5.2% of all cancer deaths. Between 2009 – 2015, the number of prostate cancer survivors over five years was 98%, which means men who have had prostate cancer treatment are living longer.[1]

Early detection and proper treatment for the stage of cancer found significantly decrease the number of deaths. Medical technology advancements have also improved greatly and should help to boost the survival rate from prostate cancer.

For various reasons, many men do not get an annual physical examination. Apparently, they do not consider their health a high enough priority. Why wait until there's pain or trouble urinating before seeing a doctor?

In my case, I had no pain or discomfort when urinating when I was told that I had prostate cancer. However, after my prostate was removed, the pathology report indicated that it was 70% cancerous.

My doctor mentioned that I was fortunate the cancer had not spread beyond the local area. If you wait until there are symptoms or pain from the prostate, the cancer may be in the third or fourth stage. In that case, the chance of survival or a complete cure is considerably lower.

My brother and I both had prostate cancer and we selected different methods of treatment. He selected radiation; I selected the radical prostatectomy.

After talking with my brother, I felt that the traditional radical prostatectomy was a much better choice of treatment for my prostate cancer. I've had fewer problems after surgery than he had after radiation treatment. It is important to ask your doctor which treatment option will be best for you, your lifestyle, and your circumstances.

1. IMPORTANCE OF EARLY DETECTION

My job required that I occasionally ride U.S. government surface ships and submarines during sea tests of new sonar systems or improvements to existing sonar systems. As a result, I was required to have an annual physical performed by a Navy doctor. I believe that annual exam saved my life.

In February 1994, a Navy Medical Officer examined me, and suggested that I see a urologist because there was something wrong with my prostate. At that time, I was employed as a civil service federal employee by the Naval Undersea Warfare Center in New London, Connecticut.

I made an appointment with my primary doctor, and he examined me and gave me a referral to see a urologist. My blood was drawn for the PSA (Prostate Specific Antigen) screening, a crucial diagnostic indicator.

Results revealed my PSA was above 4.0 (a threshold for action) and the doctor called me to schedule a biopsy of my prostate. Two days later, he called with the results: I had prostate cancer. I took a deep breath to deal with what felt like a gut punch.

But what if the doctor was wrong? I called my insurance company to find out if they would pay for a second opinion. Their answer was yes.

Later, I called my brother in California who had a high school classmate who became a surgeon. That doctor suggested I meet the Head of Urology at Yale Hospital in New Haven, Connecticut. Thankfully, I was able to get an appointment. After a review of my records and a physical examination, he confirmed that I had prostate cancer. I asked about available treatments and which options would give me more longevity. His reply was I would live longer if I had a radical prostatectomy, which in 1994 was the most advanced treatment available. He agreed to perform my surgery.

Today, there are several treatment options[2], including the following:

- Watchful waiting or active surveillance
- Surgery

12

- Radiation therapy and radiopharmaceutical therapy
- Hormone therapy
- Chemotherapy
- Biologic therapy
- Bisphosphonate therapy

Some men may require a combination of treatments. Please consult your doctor on treatment(s) that may be best for you.

I consulted two additional physicians about the best options. Without hesitation, they agreed that radical prostatectomy would give me a longer life. Don't be afraid to get second and third opinions.

From my experience, I learned the **IMPORTANCE OF EARLY DETECTION**. I have survived that deadly cancer for more than 25 years. I have dealt with many related medical problems since my surgery, but the important thing is that I'm still here to deal with these problems.

A. KNOW WHAT QUESTIONS TO ASK

It is important to be prepared for your doctor's appointment. Prior to making an appointment with my doctor to discuss treatment options, I was advised to bring a list of questions to ask along with a pad to write the answers. Some doctors also advise that you have a family member or friend accompany you to the appointment. Here's what I asked:

1. Based on my PSA, do I need a biopsy?
2. If my biopsy comes back positive, can you tell what is the stage of my cancer?
3. What is my Gleason score?
4. What treatment options are available for my stage of cancer?
5. How many patients have you treated with my stage of cancer?
6. How successful have you been in curing the cancer?
7. What are the side effects of the treatment option recommended?
8. How long after treatment would the cancer be undetectable by standard tests?

With answers to these questions, I was able to decide the best treatment option for me: the radical prostatectomy.

B. FUNCTIONS OF PROSTATE GLAND[3]

The prostate gland is a very important part of the male reproductive system. It is a small gland about the size of a walnut and is located just below the bladder and in front of the rectum. The urethra tube passes through this gland and carries urine from the bladder to the penis.

In addition, the prostate gland secretes semen that is passed through small pores of the urethra's walls during ejaculation. Moreover, there are seminal vesicles that are attached to the prostate and they provide secretions to the semen.

Sperm is manufactured by the testicles, which also produces testosterone (a male sex hormone). This hormone controls the prostate's growth and function. Therefore, the main function of the prostate is to produce fluid for semen.

C. THE GLEASON SCORE

After your doctor performs a biopsy on your prostate (the removal of prostate cells or tissues), he sends the sample to a pathologist to be examined under a microscope. The pathologist looks at the pattern of cells in the prostate tissue and grades them on a scale from 2 to 10. The most common pattern is given a grade of 1 (most like normal cells) to 5 (most abnormal).[3]

If there is a second most common pattern, the pathologist gives it a grade of 1 to 5 and adds the two most common grades together to make the Gleason score. A high Gleason score (such as 10) means a high-grade prostate tumor. These high-grade tumors are more likely than low-grade tumors to grow quickly and spread. [3]

Your Gleason score will also place you in a Grade Group[3].

- Grade Group 1 is a Gleason score of 6 or less.
- Grade Group 2 or 3 is a Gleason score of 7.
- Grade Group 4 is a Gleason score 8.
- Grade Group 5 is a Gleason score of 9 or 10.

I had a 12-core tissue sample taken during my biopsy. My Gleason score was 8, which put me in Grade Group 4 - and indicated that it was a high-grade tumor.

D. STAGES OF PROSTATE CANCER

After the biopsy indicates the presence of cancer, the doctor needs to determine the stage. This information helps patients choose the best treatment option. A doctor may order one or more body scans such as bone scan, CT scan, or MRI scan. These will provide information about the extent of the cancer and help answer these questions:

1. Has it spread to lymph nodes?
2. Has it spread to your bones?
3. Has it spread to any other organs?

In simple terms, there are four stages of prostate cancer:

STAGE I: Cancer is found in the prostate only. The cancer is not felt during a digital rectal exam and is found by needle biopsy done for high prostate-specific antigen (PSA) level or in a sample of tissue removed during surgery for other reasons. The PSA level is less than 10 and the Grade Group is 1; OR the cancer is felt during a digital rectal exam and is found in one-half or less of one side of the prostate. The PSA level is less than 10 and the Grade Group is 1.[3]

STAGE II: Cancer is more advanced than in stage I, but has not spread outside the prostate. Stage II is divided into stages IIA, IIB, and IIC. [3]

Stage II is divided into stages IIA, IIB, and IIC

15

Stage IIA: Cancer is found in the prostate only. Cancer is found in one-half or less of one side of the prostate. The prostate-specific antigen (PSA) level is at least 10 but less than 20 and the Grade Group is 1; OR cancer is found in more than one-half of one side of the prostate or in both sides of the prostate. The PSA level is less than 20 and the Grade Group is 1. [3]

Stage IIB: Cancer is found in the prostate only. Cancer is found in one or both sides of the prostate. The prostate-specific antigen level is less than 20 and the Grade Group is 2. [3]

Stage IIC: Cancer is found in the prostate only. Cancer is found in one or both sides of the prostate. The prostate-specific antigen level is less than 20 and the Grade Group is 3 or 4. [3]

STAGE III: The tumor has gone beyond the prostate and may have invaded the seminal vesicles but not the lymph nodes.

Stage III is divided into stages IIIA, IIIB, and IIIC

Stage IIIA: Cancer is found in the prostate only. Cancer is found in one or both sides of the prostate. The prostate-specific antigen level is at least 20 and the Grade Group is 1, 2, 3, or 4. [3]

Stage IIIB: Cancer has spread from the prostate to the seminal vesicles or to nearby tissue or organs, such as the rectum, bladder, or pelvic wall. The prostate-specific antigen can be any level and the Grade Group is 1, 2, 3, or 4. [3]

Stage IIIC: Cancer is found in one or both sides of the prostate and may have spread to the seminal vesicles or to nearby tissue or organs, such as the rectum, bladder, or pelvic wall. The prostate-specific antigen can be any level and the Grade Group is 5. [3]

STAGE IV: The tumor may have invaded the bladder, rectum, lymph nodes, bones, or other parts of the body. In this case, the prostate cancer is more advanced and is considered to be serious.

Stage IV is divided into stages IVA and IVB.

16

Stage IVA: Cancer is found in one or both sides of the prostate and may have spread to the seminal vesicles or to nearby tissue or organs, such as the rectum, bladder, or pelvic wall. Cancer has spread to nearby lymph nodes. The prostate-specific antigen can be any level and the Grade Group is 1, 2, 3, 4, or 5. [3]

Stage IVB: Cancer has spread to other parts of the body, such as the bones or distant lymph nodes. [3]

2. MY CHOICE FOR TREATMENT

After three doctors told me that radical prostatectomy would allow me to live longer, I scheduled the surgery.

I had shared my diagnosis with my then wife shortly after learning about it myself. Two months before I was to report to Yale Hospital in New Haven, Connecticut, I asked her to accompany me. However, when the date and time got closer and I reminded her, she told me she was **not** taking me to the hospital and suggested I ask a friend to take me.

That statement, along with a few other things, really hurt me. I knew then that her attitude and lack of support would result in the end of 35 years of marriage. I made up my mind that when I got back on my feet, I would get a divorce. Our marriage officially ended in 1996.

I faced this major surgery without her support or cooperation. A close friend agreed to take me to Yale Hospital. The operation was scheduled for 7:00 a.m. and I had to be there by 6:00 a.m. From East Lyme, Connecticut to New Haven was a 45-minute drive. We arrived at the hospital at 5:50 a.m. Needless to say, this was a stressful trip.

In 1994, the treatment method used for radical prostatectomy was called **Traditional Open Surgery** method. That method involved a long incision from my navel to the groin area that was between 8 to 10 inches in length.

The procedure had many disadvantages for the patient, such as:

1. Large amount of blood loss
2. Long and uncomfortable recovery time
3. Possible nerve damage
4. Urinary incontinence
5. Erectile dysfunction
6. Painful recovery

When the cancer is localized in the prostate gland, radical prostatectomy treatment is the most common. During my research, I've learned that this method of treatment has resulted in longer survival rates for men.

Today, there is a much better method of surgery for men who select the radical prostatectomy treatment option. In 1999, the daVinci surgical device was made available to qualified surgeons. To learn more about this device or qualified surgeons using it in your area, visit davincisurgery.com .[4] This device and type of surgery have benefits over the old Traditional Open Surgery method of prostate surgery.

I was expected to be in the hospital for five days. One day before my scheduled discharge, I had a sharp pain in my right lung when I took a deep breath. I rang the call bell, and when the nurse arrived, I described these symptoms. She performed an EKG to check my heart and confirmed I was not having a heart attack.

Shortly thereafter, I received an MRI (magnetic resonance imaging) and the results showed a blood clot in my right lung. I was told not to turn over because the blood clot would move and could cause serious problems. Later, I was taken back to my room and given blood-thinning medication to dissolve the clot.

My blood was tested every four hours to check its density. After ten days in the hospital, I was discharged. I recuperated for 30 days at home.

When I returned to work, I started thinking about retirement. I was 60 years old and had completed 39 years of federal government service. I did not have the strength to continue traveling all over the world aboard submarines and climbing ladders as my position required. In August 1994, I submitted paperwork and set my retirement date for September 23, 1994.

I visited my surgeon several times for post-op check-ups. He told me that the pathology study of my removed prostate was 70 percent cancerous, but it had not spread beyond the local area. Therefore, I did not need chemotherapy treatment. I was delighted to hear that news.

Once each month for three months, I went to Yale Hospital to meet with several urologists who asked questions about my treatment and adjustment to the side effects of the prostate surgery. I found those meetings very helpful and informative. There were several other men present during these meetings who also had prostate cancer or other urological problems. All attendees could ask any questions they wanted pertaining to their operation or adjustment after surgery.

During the first eight years following my prostate cancer surgery, I had a blood test for PSA level each year and the results were undetectable. However, sometime during the eighth year, my PSA level started rising.

My doctor monitored the rate of increase and when the PSA reached 1.0 level, I received injections of a hormone, Lupron Depot 75 mg. I then began having my PSA tested every four months, so the doctor could get an idea of the effect of the Lupron Depot injections. I received injections every four months for one and half years before my PSA became undetectable again.
After one year of being undetectable, my PSA started going up again. This up-and-down cycle of my PSA levels continues even to this day.

3. PROSTATE SURGERY SIDE EFFECTS

There are some side effects associated with radical prostatectomy. I experienced some nerve damage, incontinence (bladder leakage) and impotence (erectile dysfunction).

NERVE DAMAGE

I left the hospital with an internal catheter that had a leg bag to collect and hold urine attached. The bag remained in place for one month. When it was removed, I discovered that I was not getting a signal from the bladder to my brain that my bladder was full and needed to be emptied.

I called my doctor and explained the problem. He suggested that I try to void every two hours. This problem lasted for three months before I got a signal to my brain that my bladder was full and needed to be emptied. This experience indicated that I had some nerve damage during the surgery.

Bladder leakage was a continuous problem, and I had no control over it. I initially started wearing Depends® or undergarments to catch the urine leakage. However, soon I realized that I needed to look for a different solution for this problem because I was replacing the undergarments every two hours.

There are several incontinence products on the market, and I've tried most of them. At that time, the best one for me was Hollister products for Male Incontinence.

4. DEALING WITH INCONTINENCE

Over the last 25 years, I've had many trials and tribulations, but through it all I've managed to keep going and keep living.

Dealing with incontinence has been quite a challenge. I left Connecticut and moved to Virginia in 1996. My new doctor recommended that I try the Male Sling operation (a procedure which positions synthetic mesh to compress the urethra) to stop my bladder leakage. I had two of those operations and both were total failures.

The operation to install the Male Sling was done by a doctor in the Virginia Urology Department at Virginia Commonwealth University (VCU). I will not mention his name. I leaked just as much **after** the surgery as I did **before** the surgery.

I've tried several male incontinence products and finally settled on products made by Hollister Company. Thankfully, these products are convenient to use and not difficult to apply.

You can get a 90-day supply of medical products from a medical supply company that your insurance will pay for. Follow these specific steps to make this happen:

1. In consultation with your doctor, make a list of the incontinence supplies you need.
2. Ask your doctor to write a prescription for the products you need for a 90-day supply.
3. Email the following information to a medical supply company or order online:

   a. The prescription from your doctor
   b. List of products you need for 90 days
   c. A copy of your medical insurance card or cards
   d. Include your name, contact information, address, and phone number.

I required the following 90-day incontinence supplies:
1. External catheter, male med, latex 32mm
2. Urinary leg bag combination set, med 19
3. Leg strap catheter universal holder, white
4. A wash bottle for cleaning the leg bag

My doctor wrote a prescription for these medical products so that I did not incur significant expenses. Over the years, Medicare and my supplemental insurance have covered the entire cost of my incontinence supplies. I list any items that are not paid by my insurance on my annual tax returns.

With today's advancements in prostate cancer treatments and technologies, my hope is that a person newly diagnosed with prostate cancer will not require these supplies nor experience the related expenses.

The following are additional medical supplies I use to manage my incontinence that are not paid for by my insurance company. These are available for purchase at any drug store:

1. Lotrimin AF (ANTIFUNGAL)
2. A+D First Aid Ointment
3. Assurance Belted Shield (30 count)
4. Depends Adjustable Underwear (18 count)

Per doctor's instructions, Lotrimin AF is applied to the head of the penis **only** to prevent fungal infection. A+D First Aid Ointment is applied over the Lotrimin AF to form a vapor barrier on the head of the penis.

IMPORTANT! Do not put the Lotrimin or A+D below the head of the penis. If you do, the catheter will not stick to the penis skin. I've found it necessary to shave the hair off my penis once per week to prevent discomfort when I remove the catheter. The catheters have glue inside to make it possible to stick to the penis skin below the head of the penis.

I am 6 feet tall, and I find it necessary to add five-inch tubing to the extension tubing with connector. Occasionally when I moved my leg a certain way, it put too much tension on the catheter and caused the catheter to come off the penis. That situation was uncomfortable because my underwear and my outer pants got wet from urine. It is always necessary to leave a loop in the extension tubing to reduce tension on the catheter.

You can get additional tubing by opening another combination pack, removing the extension tubing, and cutting off 5 inches from that tubing. I have found it is best to install the additional 5-inch tubing inline next to the leg bag.

After the catheter came off twice, I started wearing Depends over the catheter everyday as a backup to prevent wetting my clothes if the catheter came apart.

My doctor told me that the catheter should not be worn 24/7. Therefore, I remove the catheter at night and used an M9 brand cleaning solution to clean the tubing and leg bag.

Also, at night I wear Depends® or Assurance® undergarments because my bladder leaks during the night. I have no control over my bladder since my prostate surgery.

5. DEALING WITH IMPOTENCE

Impotence is also known as Erectile Dysfunction (ED). Over the years since my prostate surgery, I've had quite a challenge dealing with Erectile Dysfunction. Prior to surgery, I had no problem getting an erection. Before the surgery, I was told about the side effects of a radical prostatectomy, but I didn't think they would last as long as they have.

After prostate surgery, I've had two girlfriends who understood my problem, but that did not turn them away from me. We found alternatives to sex and enjoyed each other's company going places and doing things together. Furthermore, I enjoy dancing, having taught ballroom dancing lessons over the years to young adults and senior citizens.

There are several medical conditions found to cause impotence and they include[5];

- Heart disease
- Clogged blood vessels (atherosclerosis)
- High cholesterol
- High blood pressure
- Diabetes
- Obesity
- Metabolic syndrome — a condition involving increased blood pressure, high insulin levels, body fat around the waist and high cholesterol
- Parkinson's disease
- Multiple sclerosis
- Certain prescription medications
- Tobacco use
- Peyronie's disease — development of scar tissue inside the penis
- Alcoholism and other forms of substance abuse
- Sleep disorders
- Treatments for prostate cancer or enlarged prostate
- Surgeries or injuries that affect the pelvic area or spinal cord

My conditions are prostate surgery, prostate cancer, medications, low testosterone, hormonal treatments, and nerve damage.

24

Incontinence and Erectile Dysfunction (ED) were difficult to live with at first, but over a period, I learned to adjust and I'm glad I'm still alive.

I had longtime dream and desire to see my grandchildren graduate from high school and college and get married. Two of my three grandchildren have already graduated from high school and college.

A few years after my prostate surgery, I tried some of the medical products advertised to improve erectile function. Some of the products I tried included: Cialis, Levitra, and drug injection therapy. However, I had very little success with any of them.

My current girlfriend, who is a nurse, told me about Grape Seed Extract tablets 235 mg. There are 150 tablets in a bottle of Grape Seed Extract, and I take only one tablet per day. I've been taking these tablets for six months and I noticed that I am getting better blood circulation all over my body. Maybe there is hope for me!

There are many benefits in taking Grape Seed Extract & Resveratrol tablets. The benefits that I have noticed are:

1. Helps reduce inflammation
2. Prevents formation of plaque in arteries
3. Improves poor circulation

Since taking Grape Seed Extract & Resveratrol, I have also had less pain from arthritis in my back and shoulder. Several years ago, at age 80, I was taken to an emergency room because of chest pains. The EKG test indicated that I was not having a heart attack. A cardiologist was called in and he scheduled me for a cardiac catheterization.

The doctor's report showed that I had no blockage in my arteries, and he did not find plaque in my arteries. He concluded that my chest pain was caused by the cholesterol medication I was taking. I have stopped taking all cholesterol medication.

6. IMPORTANCE OF FOLLOW-UP AFTER SURGERY

As mentioned earlier, the eight years after my prostate surgery, I continued to see my doctor each year and he checked my PSA levels. It was undetectable each year up to the eighth-year post-surgery when my PSA showed signs of going up. My doctor then requested I have a blood test every six months to monitor any increase in PSA levels. If my PSA rose above 1.0, I'd get a Lupron Depot shot. In most cases, it took 18 months for my PSA to become undetectable. Then it would stay undetectable for one year before the PSA levels started going up again. This cycle has been going on now for several years.

As you can see from my experiences post-surgery, it is very important to follow up with your doctor consistently to stay ahead of cancer getting the upper hand. I consider good health my most important asset, and I do what is necessary to be here as long as possible.

At a post-treatment visit with my doctor in 2002, my PSA was lower than it was on the previous visit. That is a good sign since I haven't had a Lupron shot in one year and a half. I hope my PSA levels continue to decrease in the months ahead.

7. LIFE AFTER PROSTATE SURGERY

Since my prostate surgery, I've had a good life. I have adjusted to my medical problems and learned to live with them as best I can. I have a supportive family and my social life is good because I have found a wonderful young lady, Sylvia W. Johnson. She loves me and accepts me as I am with all my medical problems.

Sylvia and I travel, eat out, walk, shop, and just love being together. We dance together often. I must say, we are both excellent dancers and have been in several dance exhibitions since we started dating.

Sylvia is a Certified Nurse Assistant (I), and she has helped me with many health issues. In addition to recommending Grape Seed Extract & Resveratrol, she told me to get in the habit of reading labels on items in the grocery store and buying items with less sodium, less sugar, less cholesterol and more fiber. Also, I drink alkaline water with a PH of 8.64-9.05 daily. With her help, I lost 15 pounds in two months.

My oldest son Derrick is an avid cyclist, a master martial arts instructor, and very health conscious person. He suggested the alkaline water and showed me how to breathe properly so that I won't get tired going up steps or walking up hills. As I mentioned, I was 80 years old when I began writing this book.

Every 12 months, I see my urologist doctor to check my PSA levels. I find this necessary to stay on top of my cancer trying to come back.

8. THE RISK FACTOR

I have found it is very helpful for family members in the same bloodline to know or seek out medical information about their relatives. This information may help you understand your risk factors and give you an idea of what health problems you may have to face in the future. This, in turn, enables you to prepare accordingly.

What is a risk factor? The National Cancer Institute (NCI) defines risk factor as: "Something that may increase the chance of developing a disease."[3] Some examples of risk factors for cancer include age, a family history of certain cancers, use of tobacco products, certain eating habits, obesity, lack of exercise, exposure to radiation or other cancer-causing agents, and certain genetic changes.

By knowing your family history of cancer, you can start getting certain physical examinations earlier than typical guidelines suggest. Again, why wait until you have pain or some discomfort before you see a doctor? If you keep putting off being checked, it may be too late.

I believe that my dad had prostate problems and he did not want to tell his children. As previously stated, my brother and son have also had prostate cancer. The genetic risk factor is evidently high.

MORE SPECIFIC INFORMATION ABOUT RISK FACTORS[4]

Some risk factors have been linked specifically to prostate cancer: they can raise your chance of developing the disease. Having one or more risk factors doesn't mean that you *will* get prostate cancer. It just means that your risk of the disease is greater.

AGE: Men who are 50 or older have a higher risk of prostate cancer.

RACE: African-American men have the highest rates of prostate cancer. Their disease tends to start at younger ages and grows faster than in men of other races. Asian-American men have the lowest rates of prostate cancer.

Doctors and scientists do not know why African-American men have the highest risk of prostate cancer. This indicates that more study needs to be done on this matter.

FAMILY HISTORY: Men whose father or brothers have had prostate cancer have a 2 to 3 times higher risk of prostate cancer than men who do not have a family history of the disease. A man who has three immediate family members with prostate cancer has about 10 times the risk of a man who does not have a family history of prostate cancer.

DIET: The risk of prostate cancer may be higher for men who eat high-fat diets.

9. MY BROTHER'S EXPERIENCE WITH PROSTATE CANCER

In February 2005, my brother Carl was diagnosed with prostate cancer, at the age of 67. After the biopsy and some other tests, he was told that his Gleason score was 6 (3+3). Carl was told about the different treatment options and he selected the Proton Radiation option. At the time, he was advised that the Proton Radiation option was the most exact method of treatment for him.

The Proton Radiation treatment consisted of 44 treatment sessions of one minute each for five treatments per week. I asked Carl what side effects he noticed during and after the radiation treatment. His answer was that he had no side effects.

However, Carl mentioned that nine years after the Proton Radiation treatment, different doctors alleged that the radiation damaged his bladder to the extent that his bladder would not stop bleeding. That condition resulted in the removal of the bladder.

Carl has survived the cancer for more than 15 years. I asked Carl if he had to do this over again, what treatment option would he select. His answer was doing nothing.

When I asked him if he had any suggestions for other men who are facing prostate cancer, he said, "Look at all of the options and learn about side effects for each option. Then make your choice." He also told me that he believes that many Europeans diagnosed with prostate cancer are encouraged to do nothing.

Thank you to my brother Carl for sharing his experience with prostate cancer and giving me permission to include that information in this book.

10. HERE COMES THE ROBOT

My son Derrick, also a prostate cancer survivor, tells his story here:

I knew I was at risk and figured it was just a matter of time. I hoped it would be many years down the road. But it wasn't. On March 10, 2016, a nurse's voice on the other end of the phone clearly announced, "I'm sorry to tell you that we found cancer." Despite my preparation for the inevitable, I was still a bit shocked. I was also scared … and at the same time, relieved. No more waiting; it was time to act.

In the months before my actual diagnosis, my PSA levels rose steadily from 4.3 in August 2015 to 7.82 in February 2016. Considering my age and family history, my urologist thought I would be an ideal candidate for diagnosis and potential treatment at the National Institutes of Health (NIH) in Bethesda, Maryland. NIH is known for patient study and experimental treatment. After a review of my MRI and a consultation, I would be enrolled in a prostate tissue study.

When the nurse delivered the news, she spoke calmly as she offered a date for me to visit the hospital to discuss treatment options. But based on my own research, and years of expecting this day, I already knew my preference – I asked her how soon they could remove my prostate gland. No need for discussion, let's just get it scheduled. Although she was taken aback by my response, she told me I could be scheduled the following month. This wasn't fast enough for me, but according to the doctor, waiting a few weeks would be fine.

I chose to have a radical prostatectomy using the da Vinci technology. This is a robotic-assisted surgery first introduced in 2000. Although everyone's experience is unique, the potential benefits of the da Vinci technology were attractive to me for the following reasons[5]:

- **Faster return of erectile function (ED) than patients who have had open surgery.** I experienced NO ED.
- **Faster return of urinary continence than patients who had open within 6 – 12 months of surgery.** I experienced minor dripping for about 12 months.

- **Have less chance of being readmitted to the hospital after leaving**. I did not have to be readmitted.
- **Fewer complications after surgery compared to patients who had open surgery**. I experienced NO complications after surgery.
- **Shorter hospital stays versus those patients who had open surgery**. I was in the hospital for only 48 hours.

Leading up to the Day of Surgery

I was admitted to the NIH Cancer Center on Monday, April 18, 2016, for pre-op procedures. The surgery was scheduled for the following day. I was ready. After 20 years of expecting the cancer, I wanted my body to be in tip-top shape since I had heard that helps make recovery faster. On the Sunday morning before my surgery, I did a 35-mile bike ride at an aggressive pace along with body crunches – 150 to be exact - and 10 reps of 30 Kegel (pelvic floor) exercises. On Monday morning, I did 200 body crunches and 10 reps of 30 Kegels.

When I arrived at my hospital room, my NIH roommate was Calvin B. from Georgia; we spent some time getting to know each other and sharing our diagnoses. He traveled to and from Atlanta for several months to receive a new drug regimen designed to cure his Stage Three prostate cancer. Unlike his previous treatments, this new drug was supposed to have no side effects. He would be monitored every two weeks initially, and then after the initial treatment, Calvin would come to NIH once a year for a treatment regimen. Subsequently he would come back to NIH a few times a year for monitoring.

My pre-op procedure began with a bowel cleanse. If you've ever had a colonoscopy, you know what I'm talking about. But this "juice" was much stronger and much more thorough. I had two doses over the course of a few hours. It began working very well in about an hour. Whew! After several trips to the bathroom, I was empty. It was time to rest for the big day.

The Day of Surgery

At around 6:00 a.m., a nurse arrived to take my vital signs - 111/68 with a 45 BPM. An hour later, another nurse announced my "O.R. chariot" was on its way. I was on the gurney, ready for the ride, with my wife and father standing by to wish me well. Not so fast. Evidently there had been a scheduling error; mine would now be the second procedure, not the first. What? I felt like Miss Colombia in the 2015 Miss Universe pageant, who held her new crown for five minutes before learning it was all a mistake. I was annoyed and voiced my feelings. Next thing we knew, two new drivers arrived with a gurney. Within 20 minutes, the scheduling error had been corrected. This experience underscores the importance of advocating for yourself as a patient.

Upon arrival in the Operating Room prep room, the team reviewed the procedures with us and began sedation. Before they left, my wife Diane and dad Thomas were told that because robotic surgery is performed with the patient inverted (stomach facing up) to reduce bleeding around the area, they could expect me to have a very swollen face since all the blood would pool there. I remember saying goodbye to them. My next memory was waking up in the recovery room about 2:30 p.m.

Diane and my dad met me in the recovery room. I was still loopy from the sedation, remembering only a small portion of being in the O.R. I craved ice chips as the breathing tube had left my throat very dry.

I began to assess my body and what I was feeling. In addition to a dry throat, my vision was hazy as the anesthesia wore off. My sides were tender from the six incisions around my abdomen.

I returned to my room to rest and to receive a couple of close friends and visitors. I slept and occasionally walked the halls. I was told that I needed to get up and walk around. Walking would help the doctors assess my other body functions and expedite my recovery. The goal was to do 15 laps (approximately 1 mile) around the recovery room floor, as one of the requirements for my discharge. I did eight laps the same day of my surgery. I think it paid off to be in good shape beforehand.

33

One Day After Surgery

Pain woke me around 3:00 a.m. Wednesday and I couldn't go back to sleep. I was excited to go home later in the day. Eventually I was able to fall back to sleep, but as is the case with every hospital stay, the nurse arrives on schedule to wake me and take vitals. My readings were 117/80 with a 58 BPM. An hour later, Dr. Jason S. Sedarsky, who was part of the Prostate Cancer Removal Team, led by Dr. Peter Pinto, asked how I was feeling. I explained that I had started feeling better yesterday and had even walked eight laps around my floor several hours after surgery. She knew how badly I wanted to leave. After confirming that I was doing well, she explained that I could resume a regular diet as early as breakfast. They wanted to make sure I could keep food down. The goal was to have a breakfast, lunch, and do another eight laps around the recovery ward floor before being released. I was ready and eager to meet and exceed the challenge.

I monitored my vitals daily:

> Level of Pain (LOP)- 5 on a scale of 1-10 - mild discomfort
> Meds – Percocet and Oxybutynin Chloride – for pain and bladder
>   spasms – as needed; Sildenafil (Viagra) – for six weeks;
>   Docusate Sodium (stool softener) – twice daily
> Bowel Movement (BM)- None - just wet gas in the morning
>   and dry gas in the evening
> Food -   three meals plus snacks
> Walking -   1,957 steps (Fitbit), 8 laps around the floor

I had a good breakfast but only ate half of the food. Everything stayed down. An hour after the breakfast, the nursed asked if I had a bowel movement. No movement but plenty of gas.

After breakfast, I did eight more laps around the recovery room floor, totaling 16 laps. I was feeling better and was able to do the laps without any IV stand or support. Ericka, the shift nurse, was very personable, and offered to assist me with my shower. I just couldn't refuse (smile).

By lunch time, I was hungry again and decided to get a tastier lunch. It was not bad, but I was only able to eat half. No nausea or vomiting. By now, I was counting down the hours before I could leave. My vital signs were still a bit elevated as my body worked to repair itself after the trauma of surgery.

The First Few Days Home

Thursday - This was my first morning at home, and I had a great night sleep. Even though I still had a catheter, I was home in my own bed. I spent most of the day relaxing and continued to monitor my vitals – listed below. I captured these vitals, in Tables below, to show the drops in my level of pain and increase in strength to feeling like myself again.

Day	LOP	Meds	BM	Food	Kegels	Walking Steps
Thursday	4	Vitamins (VIT), Oxycodone, Tylenol, bladder spasm med, stool softener	None – Just Gas	3 Meals plus Snacks	None	2858
Friday	3	VIT, Tylenol, bladder spasm, Viagra	Yes – One in the AM	3 Meals plus Snacks	None	4848
Saturday	2	VIT, Tylenol, bladder spasm, Viagra, stool softener	Yes – One in the AM	3 Meals plus Snacks	None	3337
Sunday	2	VIT, Tylenol, bladder spasm, Viagra, stool softener	Yes – One in the AM	3 Meals plus Snacks	None	5055

Table 1 – First few days of vitals during the recovery process

Removal of the Catheter -

It was now seven days after my surgery, and I was feeling pretty good. I continued to monitor my vitals:

Day	LOP	Meds	BM	Food	Kegels	Walking Steps
Monday	1	Vitamins (VIT), Tylenol, bladder spasm med, stool softener	Yes - Two	3 Meals plus Snacks	None	5032

Table 2 – After removal of the Catheter

I woke up about 5:00 a.m. and was unable to fall back to sleep. I was excited knowing that my catheter was going to be removed in a few short hours.

As usual, the first order of business upon arrival at the hospital is taking vitals. My readings were 109/68 BP and 55 BPM. A few minutes later I was back with a nurse preparing to remove my catheter. He asked how I was feeling and explained what was about to happen. Before he could remove the catheter, he had to conduct a bladder capacity test. This is where they fill your bladder with 120cc of sterile water and ask you to urinate it out into a flask to measure the return. After completing the bladder fill, he asked me not to urinate but to hold it until he pulled the deflated catheter out. Once the catheter was removed, I was able to produce 200cc of fluid while stopping my urine flow three times, at his request, in the process. I passed the test. He then asked if I wanted a diaper or pad. The government-issued diaper was very big, so I chose the pad. I felt I had enough control to stay dry throughout the day.

At this point, I had new freedom and no more catheter discomfort. I drove home and rested for the remainder of the day.

First Few Days without the Catheter

Tuesday was my first day without the catheter and I felt like a new person! I no longer had to worry about a bag hanging off me or the side of the bed. I continued to take my vitals:

36

Day	LOP	Meds	BM	Food	Kegels	Walking Steps
Tuesday Feeling about 85% back to normal	0	Vitamins (VIT), bladder spasm med, stool softener	Yes - Two	3 Meals plus Snacks	None	7389

Table 3 – Days after removal of the Catheter

The first night without a catheter was interesting. I wondered if I could contain the urine flow during the middle of the night or if I would awaken in a pool of urine. During the night, I had the urge to urinate three times, and got up each time to go. It was then I knew I was in control and was going to be okay. The Kegel exercises had worked. I was nine days post-surgery.

Day	LOP	Meds	BM	Food	Kegels	Walking Steps
Wednesday Feeling about 85% back to normal	0	VIT, bladder spasm (last pill), Viagra	Noticed reddish tinge to urine stream during BM – then it went away.	3 Meals plus Snacks	None	7424

Table 4 – First night after removal of the Catheter

SEX POST SURGERY

I had heard the stories; in fact, my doctors had warned me - sex would not be quite like it was, mainly because erections aren't typically as firm as they were before prostate surgery. Sparing details, I'll sum it up by saying I had no issues whatsoever with sex. Eight days post-surgery, everything felt normal. I had come home from the hospital with a supply of (and prescription for) Viagra. What a wonderful feeling! Although my erection wasn't 100% firm at first, the sensation was about the same. The biggest difference was a climax without semen. That day marked the beginning of a new normal.

This was also the first morning I resumed daily Kegel exercises. I did ten reps of a 30 count while on my back. I also began doing the Kegel exercises while standing at the sink washing dishes.

I hoped the vertical Kegel exercise would keep my thighs from getting so big, as I experienced enlarged thighs from doing the Kegel exercise horizontally in March preparing for the surgery.

Day	LOP	Meds	BM	Food	Kegels	Walking Steps
Thursday Feeling about 85% back to normal	0	VIT, Viagra	Twice. Noticed reddish tinge to urine stream during BM – then it went away.	3 Meals plus Snacks	Yes	8224

Table 5 – Sex Post Surgery

Day	LOP	Meds	BM	Food	Kegels	Walking Steps
Friday - Feeling about 85% back to normal	0	VIT, Viagra	Twice. Noticed reddish tinge to urine stream during BM – then it went away.	3 Meals plus Snacks	Yes	7259
Saturday Feeling about 90% back to normal	0 Very mild internal dis-comfort	VIT, Viagra	Twice. Noticed reddish tinge to urine stream during BM – then it went away.	3 Meals plus Snacks	Yes	8804
Sunday Feeling about 90% back to normal	0 Very mild internal dis-comfort	VIT, bladder spasm, Viagra	Twice. Noticed reddish tinge to urine stream during BM – then it went away.	3 Meals plus Snacks	Yes	8000

Table 5A

39

Spousal Support

Even before I was diagnosed with prostate cancer, Diane had been very supportive in every step of my journey. In the years prior to 2016, I had had a few scares when my PSA levels were higher than prior visits, and biopsies were ordered. Biopsies are not pleasant, and Diane would always accompany me for support. She was just as concerned as I about my potential diagnosis, prognosis, and outcome. When my PSA numbers crossed the 4.0 threshold in 2015, Diane was assertive in researching treatment options and possible side effects. She attended most doctor visits to ensure all possible questions were asked and to avoid misunderstandings or missing any possible considerations. If you can have someone accompany you to medical appointments, I highly recommend doing so. Doctor visits can be stressful and aside from moral support, it helps to have someone else listening and asking questions.

When I began to lose confidence in my initial urologist, I wanted a second opinion. I didn't feel a wait and active-watch option was in my best interest considering my family history of prostate cancer. Diane's colleague was a prostate cancer survivor and she arranged for the two of us to meet. My discussion with Diane's coworker was to understand his prostate cancer journey. What were his side-effects post-surgery? What was his recovery period? What were his experiences during his recovery? And the list goes on. I am so grateful for Diane's energy and desire to learn more about prostate cancer. She helped me become more knowledgeable about this cancer and its possible effects. From day one of my prostate cancer experience, I knew I had a wife, friend, and partner– no matter the medical outcome, good or bad. It wasn't just me facing cancer, it was us and we were preparing to deal with the unknown.

Having Diane with me throughout my entire journey has been priceless and I know that she is in this supportive role for the long-haul. I've been blessed and am very thankful for all the love and support she has provided - before, during, and after my prostate cancer procedure. Her support was important to me and my state of mind. A positive attitude has been proven to help recovery; in my case, with Diane by my side, this was certainly true.

The Importance of a Stool Softener

My doctor prescribed a stool softener and explained that I would most likely have to take it for the rest of my life. I didn't ask too many questions at first, so I didn't really understand why I needed it, I never had constipation issues before. A few weeks later, I decided to stop taking it. Bad decision – and I now count myself among people who must learn lessons – literally speaking - the hard way.

My understanding is that the colon wall with hard stool presses against the bladder and can cause a discharge of urine as I walk. So, my experiment to stop taking the stool softener not only resulted in constipation, but slight leaking – neither were welcomed outcomes.

Again, I will spare you the details (read: it wasn't a pretty scene), and just say that a dramatic experience one uncomfortable morning included an urgent trip to CVS to purchase a Fleet enema. I ended up using the pharmacy bathroom – timing wasn't on my side – but in the end, I'm thankful everything worked out just fine. The experience was a lesson to follow doctor's orders and ask questions before deviating.

Resuming Physical Activity in 60 Days

Over those first 60 days, I continued to monitor my vitals and activities while following doctors' orders. June 19, 2016 was the magic day that I could resume physical activity. I was more than ready to resume my passion: I prepped my bike, suited up, and mounted my road bike. I wanted to do 21 miles (a familiar route from DC to Maryland and back). I called one of my cycling team friends - Stan P., who had prostate removal surgery in December 2015. Stan had not been on a bike since before his surgery because he needed an additional hernia procedure post-prostate surgery. He was glad to hear from me and agreed to ride. I was still experiencing leaking and wasn't sure if sitting on the bicycle seat would cause an increase. I carried an extra pad with me just in case. It felt so good to be on the bike again, and thankfully, I had no extra leaking. My leg muscles were a bit weaker since I hadn't ridden in two months, but my core was strong, and I did not have any problems cycling. We really enjoyed the ride, and it felt great to hang out with a fellow prostate cancer survivor.

41

After the ride, I felt amazing and had no additional leaking. I was happy that I would be able to resume a normal cycling regimen within the year. My next milestone would be to slowly increase the frequency. I would ride to work two or three days a weekly, roughly four miles each way. On the following Monday, it would be my first day cycling to work post-surgery.

Post-Surgery Quarterly Checkups

July 2016
During the first quarterly checkup, my blood was drawn, and I waited about two hours for my results. Blood draws are always scheduled for the morning, followed by a midday discussion with the doctor to review and discuss any questions. My blood work showed undetectable levels for PSA. This was good news, as it initially showed that all the cancer was removed during the surgery.

The leaking was ongoing, but it had begun to slow down. The doctor asked if I was doing the Kegel exercises. I was only doing them about every other day and using one leak pad per day. The doctor recommended that I do the exercise every day to improve results.

After June 19, I'd begun cycling to work about three days a week. A quick shower upon arrival at work, and I was ready for anything the day had to offer.

First Domestic and International Trips
In August 2016, I took my first domestic flight from Washington, DC to a conference in Los Angeles, California. I was not sure how my bladder would respond to higher altitudes. Would I have more leaking due to change in air pressure. Would I bring enough pads for the entire trip? Where should I sit? Would it be better to sit near the bathroom or aisle to avoid disturbing other passengers? I decided to sit in an aisle seat to see how the ride would affect me. Getting to the flight through the parking garage and airport terminal, I didn't experience any additional leaking from previous days. While on the flight, I also did not experience additional leaking.

When I arrived in L.A., my leaking was about the same. However, when doing excessive walking, I did experience an increase. This provided a baseline in understanding some of the limitations I'd yet to overcome during travel. Over the course of my visit, I was able to control my leaking better by making sure I took more frequent bathroom visits.

At the end of September 2016, I took my first international trip to the island of Aruba with my family. I was fortunate to have had one flight experience a month earlier and knew what to expect. However, I was not thoroughly prepared for the increased leaking from walks on the beach.

Diane and I enjoyed walking on the beach in our bathing suits, but I knew this would increase my leaking. It was not a problem when I was wearing a pad, but it did become problematic when I went in the ocean to swim and then had to walk around afterwards. Leaking pads expand when they get wet.

My Recommendation: If you plan to swim, remove the pad right before it is time to get in the water. This was not a problem for me when we were near the pool as there were restrooms nearby. However, when I was on the beach in a wet bathing suit and without a pad, it would sometimes become a problem to control leaking during the walks. The blessing was that my bathing suit was already wet so a leak of a drop or two would be concealed by the wet suit and presumably go unnoticed by others. Once I knew I was not going back in the water, I'd insert a new leak pad and my concerns would go away.

October 2016
During the second quarterly checkup, I waited more than two hours after the blood draw before getting results. The blood work, once again, showed undetectable PSA levels.

The leaking continued, but it had begun to slow down even more since the last June visit. The doctor asked if I was continuing to do the Kegel exercises. I explained that I was doing them six to seven days a week. The doctor reminded me to continue Kegel exercise every day to improve results and explained I was still within the normal leaking period. He also stated that it should begin to stop within a few months.

January 2017
The third quarterly checkup also revealed undetectable PSA levels. Good news for sure.

My leaking had slowed considerably, but I still wore a pad. I was quite diligent about the daily Kegels and this made a big difference; within the last three months, I may have missed only two days of Kegels.

Even through the winter months, I continued to cycle to work about three-days a week. (I may have mentioned how much I enjoy cycling.) I even purchased cold weather gear that allowed me to ride in temperatures as low as 32 degrees.

One Year Later
April 19, 2017 marked one year since my prostate was surgically removed along with the seminal vessel. This is significant since my level of prostate cancer was 3b. The 3b designation means the cancer was outside of my prostate but contained between the prostate and seminal vessel. Even though there was no evidence of the cancer spreading outside the prostate, the doctors took samples of surrounding lymph nodes around the prostate to ensure there was no spreading. One year later, and I'm hoping my PSA levels are still undetectable.

My Recommendation: Do the exercises prescribed by your doctors because evidence shows it helps with the recovery process. I've spoken with several other prostate cancer survivors and they have all stated that they should have done more of the Kegel exercises but chose not; they either didn't make time, their egos insisted they could do without them, or their sheer stubbornness to follow a doctor's request prevailed. The bottom line is you should do the exercises because they help, and I could a see a significant slowdown in leaking when I did the exercises daily or when I just missed a day.

April 28, 2017
I had my one-year anniversary checkup. I was feeling 110% better than the previous year. The annual review was not much different than my last

44

quarterly checkup. My vitals were normal, and I had no side effects from the surgery. EVERYTHING was working as it should. Energy levels were good, and spirits were high. My PSA levels were still undetectable.

My sex life never skipped a beat. During the first few months post-surgery, I would take the prescribed 25mg Viagra tablet about twice a week. I would usually take it the night before I thought I would have sex in the morning. However, after forgetting to take the 25mg of Viagra several nights before morning sex, I found I didn't need to take it. My ability to hold and maintain an erection was not much different than if I had taken the Viagra the morning of or the night before. I stopped taking the medication altogether.

The doctor asked if I was still wearing a pad, and I said yes, due to some minor leaking tied to certain foods and martial arts activity. The doctor thought by now there should be no more pads and no more leaking. I had been wondering the same thing. After all, I'd been doing Kegel exercises six or seven times each day and they have helped. But I also remember the doctor explained that everyone recovers differently. Although my recovery immediately after surgery was very rapid, recovery for leaking was taking longer than was typical. I was disappointed but knew it would be a matter of time before I was 100% dry all day, every day.

Turns out, I had not been going to the bathroom often enough. I would wait too long and a cough or sneeze would happen. Then I immediately knew I should have gone to the bathroom earlier. I started listening to my body more; now, when I have the urge to go, I go as soon as possible.

My Recommendation: Even though you are doing everything the doctors have asked, you still need to be patient. As I was reminded, everyone will recover differently and at different rates. Continue to exercise and be diligent in following your doctor's instructions. It will pay off in the long run.

May 2017
In May, we prepared for a ten-day family vacation. This would be my second longest flight post-surgery. It would be 18 hours in the air to Thailand and about 22 hours for the return flight. Although I was not leaking, my concern was eating spicy foods and times to wait for the bathroom on the plane. What if I don't bring enough pads? What will happen if I can't control the leaking? What about my bathing suit? All these questions were circling around in my head. But I had been following doctor's orders, so I tried to relax and not worry. I just needed patience, and of course, faith.

During the trip, I was still wearing a pad a day, not because I needed it, but as a security blanket. I was in a different country with new foods, spices, and I had no idea how my body might react to these new items. After the first three days, I adjusted well. I stayed away from hot spicy foods and drinks that would trigger leaking, such as beer, spicy cocktails, coffee, and some tea. Twice during the trip however, I had foods that were spicier than I expected. Sure enough, I started leaking. I immediately refrained from eating those foods and regained control after a few hours.

Thankfully, my leaking issues were limited to the daytime. I was able to sleep through the night, much to Diane's surprise (she almost always gets up at least once each night, and thought she'd have some company – smile).

On the last few days of the trip, I noticed that the pad was staying dry. This was a good sign that my muscle control was improved. I was happy to see that things were changing for the better. Twenty-four hours after arriving home, I decided I was going to skip the pad on my return to work.

Back to Work after Long Vacation Flights
It had been two days since returning from Thailand. I had full control of my bladder and the pad stayed dry. On the next Monday morning, like most dry mornings, I rode my bike to work. After arriving to work, I'd take a shower and head to my office. On this morning, I did not wear a pad but had one in my back pocket just in case. The morning

progressed, and I was getting the urge to go to the bathroom, I would go, and everything was fine. I had no mishaps the whole day. It seemed like my time to be pad-free had come.

A few days later, I was still going through the day without a pad. I was now at the end of the week and was able to stay in full control of my bladder. This was a turning point because now I no longer had to rely on the pad. I felt freer – what a great feeling, marking my new beginning as a prostate cancer survivor. I was now completely rid of all prostate surgery dependencies, like I was before the surgery.

My Recommendation: They say patience is a virtue. I believe this whole-heartedly. It really helped me get through myriad feelings to return to how I had been pre-surgery. Patience and time, in addition to doing prescribed exercises, are going to help you see your way through. Hopefully, you have a good family and social support system, Other prostate cancer survivors also provide invaluable support since they can relate to what you are experiencing during your recovery journey. Even though experiences vary, sharing provides a different perspective and possible options and solutions you hadn't considered. I've found that having a reasonable sense of expectations and information about what you may experience helps to reduce your anxiety about the unknown.

October 2017

It had been 1.5 years since my prostate cancer surgery. I made my routine visit to NIH to have my PSA levels measured through blood work for the doctor's appointment. I headed to the outpatient clinic on the third floor for my appointment to discuss my results with Dr. Pinto's associates. I rarely see Dr. Pinto anymore since he is so busy. I met with Charlotte, Dr. Pinto's associate.

Additionally, they tested my testosterone levels since they had not been measured since pre-surgery. My testosterone level pre-surgery was 420. Today my T-Level is 380, which is considered normal. I understand your T-level should be between 200-750. Most men in their twenties are in the 700 range. Concern would arise if my T-level drops below 200. My PSA levels were undetectable.

Two Years Post-Surgery - April 2018

My spirits were high, and I was feeling great. My prior post-surgery follow-up visits were uneventful, so I didn't expect this two-year visit to NIH to be any different. I came in early morning for my blood work but this time I was told that I did not have to stay and meet with the doctor. Since I was not having any post-surgery issues, my lab results would be made available on the secure NIH Patient Portal. I missed not talking with the doctor but was also relieved to know my recovery was not something that required the doctor's concern.

Later that afternoon, my lab results were posted on the NIH Patient Portal. Again, my PSA levels were undetectable. This was a cause for celebration. I was able to continue my life as a two-year prostate cancer survivor and counting.

Journey Summary

I've been cancer free for more than three years. I've obeyed doctors' orders and am so thankful my follow-up visits to NIH show that my PSA level is undetectable. No sign of cancer. According to my doctor, reoccurrences of prostate cancer are most likely to be within one year; thus, the more frequent checkups during that period. Since I had no issues after the first year, my checkups were every six months. Now it's been more than three years with no issues, so the visits are annual.

In September 2018, I experienced a minor setback with leaking. A few drops here and there, and I had no idea to what it could be attributed. We had moved 30 days earlier – downsizing significantly to enjoy our empty nest even more, so the last thing I wanted to think about was leaking. I started wearing pads again to prevent any embarrassing episodes. Thankfully, over the four and a half-day period the leaking reduced and eventually stopped. Whew! Candidly, I still don't know what may have been the cause. Was it the three to four oatmeal cookies with the Grand Marnier drizzle every night? (Don't tell Diane.) Or maybe the stress from the move? Or maybe not doing the 50-75 miles a week on my bike prior to the move? I'm not completely sure, but I know the leaking stopped when I started riding my bike again to work every day. (Hmmm!) I'm now doing 30 – 50 miles a week if I'm lucky. The move interrupted my weekly exercise routine. Now I have to pay attention to the breaks in my daily and weekly routines. I only wore the leak pad for about three days, but I keep them hidden in strategic locations just in case another leak occurs in my future.

My journey did not start with my diagnosis in 2016. It began in 1994, after my dad's diagnosis. For those who have a family history of prostate cancer, it's often not a matter of *if* they will get prostate cancer, it is a matter of *when* it will surface. My dad explained the need for vigilance as early as possible. I was 38 years old when I had my first PSA test and prostate cancer screening.

Your mindset is very important in helping you to prepare for your prostate cancer diagnosis and aftermath. Those who seek to understand and prepare for what is yet to come will likely have a better outcome than those who wait and see what will happen before making a move. Sadly, I know several men who've waited to get checked and lost the battle as a result. Even if they lived, they were no longer able to have a quality life.

I look at this process as adopting a chess mindset vs. checkers mindset. In the game of checkers, you wait for your opponent to make a move before determining your own. In this case, your opponent is cancer. However, in the game of chess, you are strategic, trying to think 2 – 3 moves ahead of your opponent to determine possible outcomes based on your current situation. With a chess mindset, you will have a better chance of keeping your opponent in check(mate).

For men with a family history, getting regular medical checkups is key and could make the difference between life and death and help you make decisions on how to prepare for the possibility of cancer. Your preparation may include changing the foods you eat. I loved spicy foods but gave them up because they caused leaking. I've also heard, repeatedly, that sugar feeds cancer so I'm working to cut back. (It's not easy, but I'm trying.) Other preparation could include timing your doctor's checkups, learning more about technologies and procedures available for prostate cancer treatments, and most of all establishing your support systems of people who can help you along the way.

If you feel your doctor is playing checkers with your health – taking a wait-and-see attitude - you may want to seek a second opinion IMMEDIATELY. If you choose to play checkers with your health – relying solely on holistic treatments without a proven track record of success, you may want to STRONGLY consider adding conventional treatment. The outcome of a checkers approach may lead to additional complications or death.

Earlier in my journey, I mentioned that my wife Diane's support over the past few years has been priceless. In my review of prostate cancer survivor blogs and Facebook groups, I've read about the experiences of several spouses and/or partners who are enduring the prostate cancer journey with their loved one. The emotional and psychological impact has ranged from depression to stress and even emotional distance between the husband and spouse. This is unfortunate as prostate cancer is not something that's easy to experience by yourself. Your spouse/partner is the one you should be able to lean on mentally and physically. Just the realization of knowing you have cancer is bad enough.

I've experienced two forms of support – pre-surgery support when diagnosed with prostate cancer and preparing for the best treatment option. And post-prostate cancer support – once the procedure or surgery is done, getting used to the new normal of living as a prostate cancer survivor.

Before being diagnosed with prostate cancer, Diane was very involved in understanding my PSA numbers and what they meant in terms of taking action. As mentioned earlier, she was attending doctors' visits and asking questions with me to understand what I would experience and how to prepare the next course of action. I would strongly encourage any girlfriend, spouse, or partner to actively get involved to understand what your loved one may experience. Knowing what to expect with this health challenge provided us with some peace of mind while veering into unchartered territory. Diane and my ability to confront our health challenges together as a partnership and team gave me comfort that we were going to get through this challenge and outcome – good or bad. I say *our* health challenges because it would be hard for a caring spouse to sit back and watch their husband go this mental and physically draining experience without feeling some of the same level of discomfort. My dad, unfortunately, did not have the support he needed and that still bothers him to this day. Thankfully, he now has the encouragement of a caring woman.

During and after my surgery, Diane was there every step of the way. She was up-to-speed on what to expect immediately after surgery and days to follow. It was important for Diane to know this information in case, for some reason, I reached a state where I could not communicate what I was experiencing. (I advise the importance of having health care documents in place.) Luckily for me, my recovery and body changes were just as the doctors had discussed and prepared me. My recovery, in most aspects, was faster than most as I'd made a conscious effort to prepare mentally and physically for my surgery and outcome.

I was not used to being waited on and it took me a while to embrace the fact that I just needed to relax and let nature, and Diane, do those things for me that I shouldn't be doing anyway. Men reading this: please let your spouse/partner be involved in your recovery process. Your spouse's involvement may also be therapeutic for her. In my readings, I learned of spouses who would become depressed as their husbands shut them out of their recovery process. Or, the husband would have side effects from his procedure that took a turn for the worse, making it hard for both the husband and spouse to remain positively focused. As stated earlier, everyone will have a different recovery experience. Although my experiences were very positive, a small percentage of survivors have experienced complications – some self-inflicted by not following doctors' orders and others due to infections or unexpected issues beyond their control.

Take the time for you and your partner to understand options when it comes to stages of cancer and various treatments. Use a chess mindset in the way you pursue prostate cancer education and treatments. Develop a support system of people you can talk with. And most of all, keep your family and close friends informed of your progress. Again, **NO ONE** should go this journey alone.

Much has changed in prostate cancer treatment options since my dad's diagnosis in 1994 and mine in 2016. I'm not sure what new interventions or technologies will be around in the event my sons may be diagnosed with prostate cancer. I do hope that the new research and treatments will be better to allow them to have a quality life. As my quality of life was better than my dad's, I would want my sons' to be even better, even sooner than mine. I'm blessed to say I have no complaints on my quality of life post-prostate cancer surgery.

As my father stated earlier in the book, we are not doctors, nor are we in the medical profession. Please read and learn about all possible and medically proven present-day options for prostate cancer treatments and post-procedure side effects. I'm sure after reading our stories and talking with your doctor, you may learn of newer options with better results.

The purpose of sharing of our prostate cancer journeys, side effects, and present-day quality of life is to provide straightforward, personal descriptions of what we have endured. I hope my recap of my prostate cancer story has helped you see your cancer experiences in a new light. No matter your journey, you can still have a quality life when choosing the best treatment for you and your family. And after you have gone through this experience, please take the time to share your experiences with someone else who has yet to begin or is the middle of their prostate cancer journey – like my dad did with me.

CONCLUSION

My son Derrick's experience was different from mine, and that is the case for all who've been diagnosed. After reading about so many men with prostate cancer problems or dying with this disease, I decided to write this book with my son. My hope is that some or all the information presented in this book will help men and their families to better deal with prostate cancer issues.

Having prostate cancer is a life-changing event. How you deal with your diagnosis and treatment to maximize long-term survivability is the most important thing. Sure, there were many things I had to learn in order to improve my quality of life, but I'm still here to face and deal with these problems.

My two major side effects – Incontinence and Erectile Dysfunction (ED) – were difficult for me to adjust to, but over time I've learned to live with them. I'm glad that my son didn't experience any of the issues I had. It just goes to show how technology advancements can make a huge difference.

Find your tribe and hold them close. When you're dealing with cancer, it is good to have support, loving, and caring from a partner or friend. Although I did not have that from my ex-wife, I had my sons and now I have a loving, romantic relationship, for which I'm grateful. Having someone who understands my problem and who loves me, means the world to me. Without a caring person in my life, it would be very easy for me to become depressed.

Our families' prostate cancer journey has been a long one. There are three of us: my brother, my son, and me who underwent three different prostate cancer procedures and treatments. Each of us had a different outcome, but we are all still alive to enjoy our lives. I trust that you, the reader, enjoyed this book and found useful information to better understand and deal with prostate cancer. If so, please recommend to your friends and family and write an online review to help others find it.

ABOUT THE AUTHORS

Thomas A. Butts, Jr.

My parents were in their twenties when I was born on June 26, 1934, the second son of their six children. Our parents were hard workers and very loving and caring.

When I was young, airplanes fascinated me. My dad would buy model airplane kits for me to build. Then he would take me to Brookfield Park in Richmond, Virginia to fly the airplane with guide wires.

At the park, I would tell my dad that one day I was going to fly a real airplane. He would smile and say that I was just dreaming. However, my dream came true at age fifteen. I learned to fly real airplanes at that age, and I got my solo-flying license at age sixteen. I became the youngest African American licensed pilot in the State of Virginia.

I graduated from Armstrong High School in June 1952. In September of that year, I attended the University of Illinois in Champagne-Urbana, Illinois. There, I majored in Civil Engineering and completed two years before being drafted into the U.S. Air Force, where I served for four years. While in the U.S. Air Force, I traveled extensively in Europe.

I received an honorable discharge from the Air Force in May 1959 and returned to Richmond for a few months. While in Richmond, I taught ballroom dancing for three months before moving to Brooklyn, New York. In the fall of 1959, I looked for a job in electronics. I was a radar technician in the Air Force and wanted to find something in that line of work. The Brooklyn Navy Shipyard was hiring, and I was hired there. The shipyard closed in 1965 and I was hired at Naval Undersea Warfare Center in New London, Connecticut.

While working for the Naval Undersea Warfare Center, I designed sonar systems to be installed aboard target submarines for at sea testing of sonar systems aboard surface ships or submarines. In that job, I had the opportunity to travel all over the world, and I became Test Director for Target Submarines for sea test over a period of 25 years.

54

Derrick A. Butts

I was born August 4, 1962 in Brooklyn, New York. Raised in Connecticut from age four until I went to college at North Carolina A & T State University in Greensboro, North Carolina on a Navy Cooperative Education scholarship to pursue a degree in Electrical Engineering. After college, I obtained a masters' degree in Telecommunications Management from University of Maryland University College.

I've worked at a variety of places including the same Naval Undersea Warfare Center in New London, Connecticut, as my dad. My work has always been in technology fields at companies that include Martin Marietta Aero and Naval Systems, Voice of America, MCI, Electric Lightwave, and Siemens Enterprise Communications.

I'm well-versed in enterprise business continuity design strategies, domestically and internationally, for cyber-secure infrastructures, interoperability, cloud computing, and virtual networking. In 2008, I left the corporate world to begin my own business – Continuums Corp – focused on secure business continuity strategies for enterprise architectures and consulting for the Navy DoD. In 2015, I became the Chief Information and Cybersecurity Officer (CIO/CO) for Truth Initiative, a non-profit inspiring tobacco-free lives.

Additionally, I'm a century cyclist and have been a martial arts practitioner, in over seven different styles, for more than 47-years. I hold a 4th Degree (Master Instructor) Black Belt in Tang Soo Do and Tai Chi. I live in Washington, DC with my loving wife, Diane. My two sons, Jamel and Jared, live in Brooklyn, New York.

AFTER 85 LONG YEARS, I'M STILL HERE

Each morning I wake up, I thank God for giving me another day. Life has not always been a bed of roses for me. On this journey through life, I've had many trials and tribulations, many ups and downs, and a battle with prostate cancer and two total knee replacements. Yet through it all, God has kept me here.

As a twenty-five-year cancer survivor, I feel that I have really been blessed. God helped me to survive a major fire aboard an aircraft carrier where 51 men lost their lives. Also, he helped me to realize my childhood dream to become a licensed pilot at the young age of 16 years old.

For my vocation, God helped me to get a wonderful job where I traveled almost all over the world aboard U.S. submarines as a civilian on someone else's dime. Yes, I can truly say that I've been blessed during my 85 years on this earth. I look forward too many more happy and challenging years in the future. Yes, it is wonderful to say, **I'M STILL HERE.**

Thomas A. Butts, Jr.

REFERENCES

1) National Cancer Institute, NIH, Cancer Stat Facts: Prostate Cancer – June 15, 2019 - **https://seer.cancer.gov/statfacts/html/prost.html**

2) National Cancer Institute, Prostate Cancer Treatment (PDQ®)–Patient Version – June 22, 2019
https://www.cancer.gov/types/prostate/patient/prostate-treatment-pdq

3) National Cancer Institute, NIH Publication No. 12-1576, Revised June 2012 "What You Need to Know About Prostate Cancer"

4) Why Surgery with da Vinci? - June 2019
https://www.davincisurgery.com/procedures/urology-surgery/prostatectomy

5) Mayo Clinic, Patient Care and Health Information, Diseases and Conditions – Erectile Dysfunction – July 4, 2019
https://www.mayoclinic.org/diseases-conditions/erectile-dysfunction/symptoms-causes/syc-20355776

6) National Cancer Institute, NIH Publication No. 11-4303, Reprinted August 2011 "Understanding Prostate Changes a Health Guide for Men"